Chair Yoga for Women over 40

Easy and Quick Guide for Weight Loss

Dovie Betty

Copyright © [2023] by [Dovie Betty]

All rights reserved.

No portion of this book may be reproduced in any form without written permission from the publisher or author, except as permitted by U.S. copyright law.

Table of Contents

INTRODCTION

Jessica was a woman who lived in a quiet nook of Springfield, a bustling city where life moved quickly. She was an ambitious, free-spirited woman in her early 40s with big plans and goals. Her passion for life was unshakeable, and her laughter was contagious. Beneath that bright grin, though, was a difficulty many women in their 40s can identify with: managing their weight.

Jessica had gone through the natural changes that come with time, just like many of us. The metabolism that had previously permitted excesses now appeared to be slowing down. She didn't have much time for herself because of her busy schedule. The strains of life had made her unintentionally forget the most important person in her life: herself.

Jessica had a wake-up call resonate throughout her during a regular check-up, when the doctor's remarks contained underlying worry. She began to think about herself and take action after seeing the numbers on the scale and hearing the doctor's kind comments about how important it was to maintain a healthy weight for her age. Even if it was just for a little while, she needed to get off the merry-go-round since the globe was whirling so quickly.

Jessica set out on a mission to live a happier and healthier life. As she went on her adventure, she encountered an unusual friend in the most unexpected of places—a basic chair.

Jessica's path is not unique to her; many women over 40 may relate to it. It's an empowering, self-discovery, and resilient journey. This is a voyage that blends the ordinary and the extraordinary, the profound and the practical. This trip leads us to the main destination of the book, "Chair Yoga for Women Over 40 Weight Loss."

I shall explore a holistic approach to wellbeing designed for women like Jessica in the pages that follow. I will go into the practice of chair yoga, which is an approachable and useful way to improve your health and lose weight. I welcome you to go on a journey of self-care, change, and eventually empowerment with me, guided by the knowledge found in this book.

Now, my dear reader, flip the page. Learn about Jessica's story, accept the benefits of chair yoga, and uncover the key to a happy, healthier you. Your voyage has begun.

Chapter 1: Getting Started with Chair Yoga

Setting Up Your Space for Practice

If you want to get the most out of your chair yoga sessions as a woman over 40, it's critical to create a comfortable and secure environment. I'll look at how to set up your practice area in this chapter so you can start your chair yoga adventure with confidence and comfort. Just a few changes to your surroundings may have a big impact on your practice; you don't need a sophisticated studio or a lot of room.

1. Selecting an Appropriate Location

The place you choose when you're ready to begin practicing chair yoga is crucial.
 Here are some points to think about:

Find a place that is calm and tranquil so that you can concentrate without being overly distracted. This may be a quiet bedroom, a nook in your living room, or even a designated area in your home office.

Natural light is best since it may improve your mood and make you feel more connected to your practice. Make sure the area you have picked has enough artificial lighting if there isn't any natural light available.

Make sure the place you've picked is well-ventilated. You won't feel stuffy or hot throughout your practice since there is adequate air circulation.

2. Required Resources

Although chair yoga doesn't require much gear, the following items will improve your practice:

Chair without Wheels: Select a chair that is stable. It needs to be armless and have a straight back. This gives your practice a secure and encouraging base.

Yoga Mat or Non-Slip Surface: By placing a yoga mat or a non-slip surface under your chair, you may improve its stability when performing standing postures and stop it from slipping.

Wear loose, comfortable attire that doesn't restrict your ability to move. Simply wearing anything that allows you to move and stretch freely won't do for yoga.

Bare Feet or Non-Slip Socks: When practicing chair yoga, keeping your balance is much easier by wearing bare feet or non-slip socks.

3. Safety Measures

Any yoga practice must be done safely. Observe the following key safety measures:

Clear the Area: Make sure there are no obstructions or tripping hazards around your chair. To move your arms and legs comfortably, you need an appropriate room.

Make sure your chair is sturdy by placing it on a solid surface. To prevent any wobbling, make sure that all of the chair's legs are securely planted.

Personal Limitations: Recognize your physical boundaries and work within them when practicing. Consult a medical expert or a trained yoga instructor if you have certain health issues or injuries so they may help you modify your practice.

Have a strategy in place in case you require support or help while working out, such as having a phone close by or telling a family member when you practice.

Setting up your area may seem like a little matter, but it's crucial to creating a comfortable, pleasurable, and secure environment for your chair yoga practice. You'll be better prepared to get into your chair yoga program with assurance and attention after your practice area is set up. The essential elements of chair yoga will be discussed in the following chapters, making your trip even more convenient and fulfilling.

Finding the Right Chair and Equipment

Prior to starting your chair yoga adventure, it's crucial to get the proper tools. In this chapter, I'll go into more depth on selecting the ideal chair and other necessary pieces of gear to make your chair yoga practice secure, cozy, and productive.

Selecting the Ideal Chair

Your practice of chair yoga is built on the chair you choose. Observe the following:

Stability Is Important

Find a chair that is reliable and solid. Its surface needs to be level and even, and all of its legs ought to be securely planted. Your safety while practicing should be ensured by the chair not rocking or tilting.

Seat Depth and Height

When you are sitting comfortably, the ideal chair should have a seat height that enables your feet to rest flat on the floor. Think about the seat's depth as well. Choose a chair whose seat is not too deep so that you may rest your back on the backrest without having trouble sitting up straight.

3. Back Support and Armrests

For balance and support during chair yoga postures, armrests might be useful. A chair with a firm backrest can also help in maintaining good posture and easing tension.

4. Slip-Proof Surface

Make sure the seat and back of the chair are non-slip or have a non-slip cover. This stops you from slipping when doing chair yoga.

5. Comfort and Protection

You want stability, but you also want to be comfortable. Pick a chair with enough padding to make practicing comfortable.

6. Room for Motion

Take into account the area around the chair. Yoga positions should be performed in an unobstructed space with ample space.

Getting More Equipment Together

A few extra pieces of equipment, in addition to the chair, can improve your chair yoga practice:

Yoga Mat or a Non-Slip Surface

To keep your chair from shifting while you practice, place a yoga mat or other non-slip surface under it. This creates an additional level of security.

2. Blocks and Cushions

Use additional cushions or yoga blocks to increase the comfort of your practice if the seat or back of your chair isn't well-cushioned.

Bands of resistance

Your chair yoga exercises might benefit from the versatility of resistance bands. For workouts that increase strength, they serve as resistance.

4. An alarm or timer

Setting a time restriction for your chair yoga practices with a timer or alarm will help you stay consistent.

5. Bottle of water

Keep yourself hydrated while you practice. Keep a water bottle close by hand so you may sip as necessary.

6. Relaxed Clothes

When practicing chair yoga, dress in comfortable, loose-fitting attire that allows for effortless mobility.

It could take some effort to find the proper chair and equipment, but doing so is an investment in your health and wellbeing. When everything is set up just so, you can start practicing chair yoga with assurance. The next chapters will cover a variety of topics to aid you in your weight reduction quest, including breathing exercises and fundamental chair yoga positions.

Chapter 2: Chair Yoga Basics for Beginners

Breathing Techniques for Relaxation and

Energy

A crucial component of yoga is breathing, and learning to control your breath in chair yoga for weight reduction may be game-changing. I'll examine the enormous effects that mindful breathing may have on energy and relaxation in this chapter. As a foundation for your chair yoga practice and weight reduction quest, you'll discover useful breathing methods that are practical and advantageous for women over 40.

The Study of Breathing

It's essential to comprehend the science behind breath and how it impacts our body and mind before we get into the practices. Our neural system and respiratory pattern are tightly related. While slow, deep breathing activates the relaxation response, shallow, fast breathing can set off the body's stress reaction.

Start with the fundamentals by using diaphragmatic breathing. Put one hand on your chest and the other on your belly while sitting comfortably in your chair. Allow your abdomen to expand as you inhale deeply through your nose before gently exhaling through your mouth. As you do this, feel your shoulders and chest unwind. You can relax more and feel less stressed with this method.

Relaxation Breathing

Let's look at how regulated breathing may encourage relaxation because stress and tension can be obstacles to losing weight.

4-7-8 Breath: This method is straightforward but efficient. Breathe in via your nose for four counts, hold it for seven counts, and then let it out through your mouth for eight counts. With your attention on your breath and the counting, repeat this cycle many times. It is an efficient way to quiet down your nervous system.

Alternate nostril breathing involves gently pinching one nostril shut with your thumb while breathing in through the other. Exhale through the first nostril while covering the other nose with your ring finger. This cycle encourages tranquility and equilibrium.

Take a Breath for Energy

Having enough energy is crucial for being active and promoting weight reduction. By using these strategies, you may increase your energy while doing chair yoga.

Sit up straight, take a big breath in, and then forcefully expel through your nostrils to do the breath. Pay attention to the exhale. Your energy and mental clarity may improve with this quick exhalation method.

The technique Breath is frequently referred to as the "ocean breath." Create a quiet, audible sound by inhaling through your nose, tightening your throat, and gently exhaling through your nose. It's a fantastic method to revitalize and warm up your body before doing chair yoga.

Chair yoga with breath included

Let's look at how to incorporate some helpful breathing exercises into your chair yoga practice now that you've learnt them.

Chair yoga postures should be performed while breathing in harmony with your movements. When stretching or extending, inhale; when contracting or relaxing, exhale. This helps you stay rooted and maximizes the advantages of your yoga and breath exercises.

Breath Awareness: Throughout your practice, pay close attention to your breath. Do you have regular, deep breathing? To keep yourself calm and focused during your session, follow the cues of your breath.

Simple yet effective breathing exercises will improve your chair yoga practice and help you achieve your weight reduction objectives. You'll discover that by implementing these practices into your daily life, you'll experience more energy and relaxation as well as a closer connection to your body and mind. A major component of chair yoga is breathing, which you may practice on your way to greater health and wellbeing.

Seated Warm-Up Exercises

It's crucial to begin with a moderate warm-up before beginning your chair yoga adventure. You may prepare your body for a successful and secure chair yoga practice by performing these sitting warm-up movements. Women over 40 should specifically focus on warm-up activities since they reduce the risk of injury, increase circulation, and ease you into your practice. I'll walk you through a variety of sitting warm-up exercises in this chapter that are intended for those just starting out on their weight-loss journeys.

Why Warmup Is Important

Every yoga practice should begin with a good warm-up to get your muscles and joints ready for movement. Why it's crucial for women over 40 is as follows:

Preventing injuries: As we become older, our bodies may be more prone to sprains and injuries. By prepping your muscles and joints, a warm-up helps lower this danger.

Improved Circulation: By getting your blood moving during chair yoga warm-up movements, your muscles and organs will receive more oxygen and nutrients.

Increased Flexibility: By improving joint mobility with gentle warm-up stretches, you may more easily transition into challenging positions.

Mental Preparedness: Warming up aids in the transition from the stresses of daily life to the focused practice of yoga.

Warm-up exercises while seated

1. Neck ties

Gently rotate your neck in a clockwise and counterclockwise direction. For individuals who spend a lot of time sitting at a computer, this exercise is especially good since it relieves neck stress.

Rolling the shoulders

Straighten your spine and shrug your shoulders back and forth. This exercise improves posture while releasing stress in the shoulders and upper back.

3. Hand Circles

Make mild wrist motions in both directions as you extend your arms out in front of you. Carpal tunnel syndrome and wrist sprains are both prevented by this workout.

Fourth, Ankle Circles

Rotate your ankles clockwise and counterclockwise while raising one leg at a time. The lower legs' circulation is enhanced, and the workout encourages ankle flexibility.

5. Cat-Cow Stretch while seated

Put your hands on your knees and sit back in your chair. In the "Cow Pose," you inhale, arch your back, and elevate your chin. In the "Cat Pose," take a breath round your pelvis, and tuck your chin. To warm up your spine and encourage flexibility, perform this movement repeatedly.

6. Light twists

Place your feet firmly on the floor while sitting on the edge of your chair. Gently turn to the right while placing your left hand on your right knee. After a few breaths of holding, transfer sides. Twisting stretches aid in spinal decompression and internal organ massage.

7. Deep Inhalation

Sit up straight, close your eyes, and concentrate on your breathing. Breathe in deeply and slowly, using your nose to inhale and your mouth to exhale. Deep breathing helps to relieve tension, quiet the mind, and get you ready for your yoga practice.

Each of these chair yoga warm-up movements is appropriate for women over 40 and offers a gentle, powerful method to get your body and mind ready for the practice. Keep in mind to walk gently and deliberately while paying attention to your body's cues. As you move toward your weight reduction objectives, these exercises lay the groundwork for a secure and fulfilling chair yoga practice.

Building Strength with Chair Poses

You're invited to go on a journey of strength-building using the gentle but effective technique of chair yoga. The desire for fitness presents special difficulties for women over 40. I will examine how Chair Yoga may help your efforts to lose weight, improve muscle tone, and develop strength in this chapter. Learn how simple chair postures have the ability to alter your body and mind.

Chair Yoga: A Foundation for Strength

Understanding the Chair Yoga's Fundamental Strength:
In the realm of yoga, developing functional strength, flexibility, and balance is just as important as lifting heavy objects. For women over 40, Chair Yoga offers a strong foundation for building strength in a kind, useful, and long-lasting manner.

Examine the details of muscle activation using chair poses. Engaging Key Muscle Groups. Discover which muscle areas each posture targets, boosting strength without undue effort. Learn how these positions affect total muscle tone and body awareness from the core to the arms.

Chair Pose Development for Specific Strength Training

Explore the subtleties of the fundamental position seated mountain stance, which engages the core muscles, for core stability. Recognize how this basic sitting position encourages stability, improves posture, and paves the way for more challenging postures that develop strength.

Explore the mechanics of Chair Squats, a dynamic stance that focuses the lower body, for greater lower body strength. Discover the advantages for the glutes, hamstrings, and quadriceps when sitting still. To adjust the intensity to your level of fitness, learn variants.

Discover the powerful qualities of seated warrior poses, which are intended to strengthen the arms and shoulders. Learn the right posture and strengthening methods for your upper body to improve your ability to do everyday tasks with ease.

Developing Your Chair Yoga Strength Program

Creating a Custom Strength-Building program: Instructions on how to design a Chair Yoga program that meets your specific requirements and objectives. Learn the fundamentals of sequencing to develop a balanced practice that gradually increases strength over time.

Strength-Building Activities to Include in Daily Life: Find out how to include Chair Yoga strength training into your regular practice. Learn how a few short, regular workouts may help you build strength over time.

Strengthening with Intention for Women Over 40

Examine the significance of maintaining a balance between strength and flexibility. Discover how Chair

Yoga promotes both, improving general mobility and lowering injury risk as you age.

Strength Training and the Mind-Body Connection: Chair Yoga is a great way to explore the mind-body connection part of strength training. Recognize how mindfulness improves the efficacy of your practice and fosters overall wellbeing.

It's important to keep in mind that even the smallest effort may result in substantial advancement as you set out on your Chair Yoga strength-building adventure. Recognize the transforming impact these poses pose for women over 40 on their weight reduction and health journeys, and embrace their simplicity and accessibility.

Make strength more than simply a physical quality; make it a constant companion in your life.

Balance and Flexibility for Everyday Life

Welcome to the section on using chair yoga to increase your flexibility and balance. Balance and flexibility are crucial to achieving and maintaining on our path to weight loss. These characteristics become increasingly more crucial for daily living as we become older. We'll explore the significance of balance and flexibility, how they affect your attempts to lose weight, and how chair yoga can help you improve these areas of your health in this chapter. Because we want to make this accessible to everyone, especially women over 40, we'll keep the terminology clear and uncomplicated.

The Importance of Flexibility and Balance

Balance and flexibility are the unsung heroes of your body. Though they might not receive as much emphasis as weight loss or strength training, they are just as important to your general health.

Balance: Maintaining your equilibrium helps you avoid falls, which can be particularly dangerous as we age. It's important to avoid injuries in addition to being sturdy on your feet. Being balanced makes it simpler to walk around with confidence, participate in physical activity, and maintain an active lifestyle. You can accomplish your weight loss goals thanks to this.

Regarding flexibility, range of motion is everything. You can bend over, tie your shoes, and reach for objects with it without exerting yourself or getting hurt. Daily tasks become simpler and exercise is more effective when you are more flexible. Additionally, it might aid in easing the aches and pains that occasionally occur with aging.

Chair yoga promotes stability and flexibility

Let's now discuss how chair yoga can improve your flexibility and balance. Given that it takes into account your unique demands and challenges, it is ideal for women over 40.

Chair yoga is a form of classical yoga that has been modified for seated positions. This makes it safe and convenient for everyone to practice balance and flexibility without having to sit on the floor.

Stretching gently: Chair yoga involves stretching gently, which helps to increase flexibility. Your range of motion will progressively expand, making daily activities easier.

Strengthening the core: Balance requires a strong core. Core-strengthening movements are incorporated into chair yoga to assist you maintain stability while sitting and moving.

Breathing and mindfulness are two aspects of chair yoga that are frequently emphasized. These aspects can help you maintain concentration and calm while practicing your balance.

Chair yoga: Including It in Your Routine

Consider these useful suggestions to get the most out of chair yoga for increasing flexibility and balance:

Key is consistency. Aim for consistent practice, even if it just lasts a short while each day.

Be aware of your body. Modify or skip a pose or stretch if it hurts or feels uncomfortable.

To help you with your practice, use props like a belt or a cushion. Pose accessibility may be increased by these.

Challenge yourself gradually. Try more difficult chair yoga poses and stretches as you get more at ease.

Remind yourself to breathe. The advantages of chair yoga are enhanced by deep, focused breathing.

Always keep in mind that growth takes time, so have compassion on yourself. You'll eventually develop better flexibility and balance.

For balance and flexibility, chair yoga is not only a useful but also a wise addition to your regimen. By simplifying daily tasks and encouraging activity, it aids in your weight loss efforts. So sit down in a quiet area, grab a chair, and let's practice balance and flexibility for a healthier, more agile you.

Chapter 3: Crafting Your Chair Yoga Routine

Creating a Personalized Chair Yoga Plan

Personalization is your hidden weapon in the fight to reach your weight reduction objectives with chair yoga. Because each body is different, what fits one person may not be the greatest for another. We'll explore the craft of developing a customized chair yoga schedule that is made just for you in this chapter.

Recognizing Your Needs

Let's first determine your specific demands before creating your own chair yoga regimen. Your age, level of fitness, weight reduction objectives, and any physical restrictions are all important factors in creating a strategy that works for you.

How to Evaluate Your Fitness

Start by evaluating how fit you are right now. It's okay if you're new to chair yoga or haven't been physically active in a while. Your strategy might begin where you are now and advance gradually.

Realistic Goal Setting

Setting attainable weight reduction goals is crucial. Regarding your goals, be clear-cut and practical. For instance, defining specific goals that can be achieved in a fair amount of time is more doable than having general targets.

Consider your physical restrictions.

Be mindful of any physical restrictions or health issues you may have. Due to its adaptability, chair yoga is appropriate for those with a variety of physical ailments. Your strategy can be altered to meet your specific requirements.

How to Create a Chair Yoga Routine

It's time to create your customized chair yoga regimen after evaluating your demands.

Selecting Appropriate Pose

Choose chair yoga positions that support your objectives. Include stretches and mild twists if you want to increase flexibility. Include positions that work your muscles if building strength is your goal.

Conversion for Comfort

Make sure you feel at ease in the postures you select. Investigate changes or skip a position if it doesn't feel correct or causes pain. Your chair yoga program should encourage wellbeing rather than agony.

Cardio and relaxation in harmony

The key is balance. Include heart-raising chair yoga routines to improve your cardiovascular health. Combine them with exercises that support awareness, stress reduction, and relaxation.

Advancement and Variety

Monitoring Your Development

Record your chair yoga sessions and the amount of weight you are losing. Examine your energy levels, mood, and any physical changes on a regular basis. This will assist you in maintaining motivation and making the necessary changes to your strategy.

Establishing Variety

Introduce variation to avoid becoming complacent and plateauing. Regularly switch up your chair yoga practices. Examine various teachers, positions, and sequences. This will keep your work exciting and novel.

Be flexible and attentive to your body.

Above all, keep in mind that your customized chair yoga plan is a dynamic guide. Be prepared to modify your strategy if you experience setbacks or changes in your life. Pay attention to and heed your entire body's messages.. It may be wise to relax for a day or two from time to time.

Chair yoga personalization is a journey that changes as you do. As you hone your strategy to be uniquely you, have patience and kindness for yourself. To make sure that your individualized plan turns into a powerful tool in your quest for wellbeing, we'll go deeper into chair yoga sequences and tactics that are tailored to your weight reduction objectives in the chapters that follow.

Sample Chair Yoga Routines for Weight Loss

I will get into the use of chair yoga for weight loss in this chapter. I'll look at a few sample chair yoga practices made just for ladies over 40. These exercises are intended to be simple, pleasant, and useful. They will complement your weight reduction efforts and help you increase your metabolism and flexibility. Let's get started with chair yoga, which is all about making things simple and pleasurable.

Chair Yoga Exercises for Weight Loss Examples

Routine 1 of Chair Yoga: Energizing Morning Sequence

Setting a good tone for the remainder of the day with an energized chair yoga session might be beneficial. This series emphasizes on slow, relaxing motions that awaken both your body and mind.

1. Tadasana, or seated mountain pose

Put your feet firmly on the ground and sit up straight. Reaching out toward the ceiling, raise your arms in the air.
Take a big breath in and raise your body.

Breathe out as you gradually lower your arms.
2. Cat-Cow Stretch while seated

Put your hands on your knees and sit up straight.
In the "Cow Pose," inhale, arch your back, and look upward.
Take a breath out, arch your back, and chin-tuck to your chest (cat stance).
Set your breath in time with your movement as you go through this flow multiple times.
3. Sit-Facing Fold

Put your feet flat on the ground and lean back in your chair.
Expand your spine as you inhale.
As you slowly stretch forward toward your feet while exhaling, hinge at the hips.

Feel the stretch in your back and hamstrings as you hold for a few breaths.
4. Sitting Twist

Put your right hand on the outside of your left knee while sitting up straight.
Expand your spine as you inhale.
Take a breath out, turn to the left, and glance over your left shoulder.
Hold for a few breaths before transferring to the opposite side.
This practice is ideal for a hectic morning because it can be completed in only 10-15 minutes. It aids in waking up your body, improving blood flow, and setting a good mood for the day.

Mid-Day Stress Buster: Chair Yoga Routine 2

This chair yoga exercise will help you unwind and re-energize when you need a break in the middle of a busy day.

1. Sun Salutation while seated

Put your feet firmly on the ground and sit up straight.
As you exhale, lift your arms in the air.
Reaching for your toes while exhaling forward.
Exhale to drop your arms as you inhale to stand up straighter.
Sitting Warrior two.

Place your right foot on the ground and stretch your left foot back as you sit at the edge of your chair.
With your palms facing down, lift your arms to shoulder height.

Breathe out, bending your right knee just a little, look over your right hand.

3. Tree Pose when seated

Put your hands on your hips and sit up straight.
Lift your right foot to rest on your left calf as you inhale.
As you establish your equilibrium, hold for a few breaths.
Change to the opposite side.

4. Relaxation and deep breathing when seated

Place your hands on your lap while you sit comfortably.
Take a few calm, deep breaths while closing your eyes.
Concentrate on calming your body and releasing tension and stress.
This mid-day ritual helps you relax, think more clearly, and have more energy. During your lunch break or any

other free time during the day, it may be finished in only 15-20 minutes.

Chair Yoga Routine #3: Evening Stretch and Relaxation

This chair yoga exercise encourages relaxation when the day comes to an end, helps reduce muscular tension, and gets your body ready for a good night's sleep.

1. Pose of a seated child

Bring your knees close together as you sit up straight.
As you lean forward and lay your chest on your thighs, inhale and then exhale.
Put your forehead on your crossed arms while extending your arms forward.
2. Sitting Leg Extensions

One leg should be extended while you sit at the edge of your chair.

Take a deep breath in, stretch your back, and gradually hinge over your extended leg.

Then, move to the other leg after holding for a few breaths.

3. Pose of the Seated Pigeon

Cross your right ankle across your left knee while sitting up straight.

To feel a stretch in your hip, gently press down on your right knee.

Hold for a few breaths before transferring to the opposite side.

4. Deep breathing while relaxing on a chair

Place your hands on your lap while you sit comfortably.

Take a few calm, deep breaths while closing your eyes.

Concentrate on letting your body relax and become less tense.
Your muscles will relax as a result of this nighttime ritual, and you'll feel calmer. It's a great way to round up the day and get ready for a restful night's sleep.

Keep in mind that you may adjust and personalize these chair yoga practices to meet your requirements. The secret is to exercise frequently, maintain consistency, and pay attention to your body. You'll eventually notice how chair yoga helps your efforts to lose weight.

Staying Consistent with Your Practice

I'm going to examine one of the most important components of your chair yoga and weight reduction journey in this chapter: consistency. It's simple to become excited when you first start, but consistency over time is what yields real results. We'll look at useful techniques to help you stay motivated, create realistic objectives, and get past typical roadblocks that might impede your development.

Realistic Goal Setting

Consistency is based on setting attainable goals. Think about the following when doing chair yoga for weight loss:

Make sure that your objectives are S.M.A.R.T. (Specific, Measurable, Achievable, Relevant, and Time-bound). Instead of stating a general objective like "losing weight," for instance, say you aim to "lose 1 pound per week for the next 10 weeks."

Break your trip into more achievable, short-term, and long-term milestones. Long-term objectives offer you direction, while short-term goals give you a sense of success.

Flexibility: Make room for modifications. It's okay when life gets in the way from time to time. Be prepared to modify your objectives if necessary.

Establishing a Reliable Routine

Chair yoga should be a part of your everyday ritual. This habit will help your practice feel more natural, even if it's just for a short while.

Scheduled Sessions: Make a timetable for your chair yoga sessions and follow it. Knowing your practice schedule will enable you to prioritize it.

Partner up with a friend or family member as your accountability partner to practice or check in on each other's progress. You can stay motivated if you have accountability.

overcoming obstacles

Plateaus and boredom: Change things up if you start to become weary of your routine or you see a halt in your weight reduction. Try out new chair yoga poses, mix up your routine, or get ideas from other teachers.

Injury and Pain: If you're experiencing pain or injury, don't let that deter you. Make adjustments to your chair yoga exercise to suit your needs, and seek medical advice if required.

Time Restrictions: Life may become busy, but chair yoga can always fit into spare moments. Even a little session of 10 minutes might be helpful. Keep in mind that consistency matters more than time.

Encouragement and self-care

Find out what motivates you to practice chair yoga using our motivation toolbox. It may be keeping track of your progress, feeling more energized, or enjoying the process. Keep a toolbox of inspiration in your possession.

Don't underrate the importance of taking care of yourself. To refresh your body and mind, use relaxation techniques like deep breathing, meditation, or mild stretches.

Community and Assistance

Joining a Group: Take into account signing up for a chair yoga session or a group of like-minded people online.

Making people aware of your trip may increase motivation and create a support network.

Recognize and appreciate your successes, no matter how modest they may be. Your confidence and devotion are strengthened by small victories.

The key to success in chair yoga for weight reduction is consistency. You'll be well on your way to losing weight and feeling your best if you set reasonable objectives, establish a regular practice schedule, overcome obstacles, stay motivated via self-care, and seek out community and support. Keep in mind that progress, not perfection, is the goal.

Chapter 4: Yoga for Weight Loss

Understanding How Yoga Supports Weight Loss

Yoga, a timeless old discipline, provides a comprehensive approach to health and well-being. In this chapter, I'll look at how yoga, and more especially chair yoga, might help an older woman who is trying to lose weight. Let's explore the science and application of chair yoga to get rid of those excess pounds and transform into a healthier, happier you.

Recognizing Yoga's Support for Weight Loss

Yoga isn't about making yourself into a pretzel or breaking a sweat in a heated environment. Instead, it's a kind and long-lasting way to lose weight, especially for women over 40.

1. Mind-Body Connection: The Secret to Long-Term Loss of Weight

Yoga is all about harmony, and this applies to your weight as well. Your mind and body are connected, increasing your awareness of your body's requirements. Effective weight control requires this kind of attentiveness. By promoting slow, controlled movements and deep, mindful breathing, chair yoga helps people connect.

2. Increased Metabolism: Gracefully Burn Calories

Our metabolism frequently slows down as we become older, making it more difficult to lose weight. But chair yoga increases your metabolism. You activate different muscle areas with these mild motions, which increases calorie burning. It's a quiet yet powerful approach to boost your metabolism without overworking your body.

3. Stress Management: Say Goodbye to Emotional Eating

Life may be challenging, particularly for active women over 40. Emotional eating and weight gain are frequently caused by stress. You may control your stress by doing chair yoga, which has a relaxing effect on the mind. It gives you the ability to address the underlying reasons of overeating through deep relaxation methods and meditation.

4. Lean and Strong Muscle Development

Contrary to popular belief, muscle is more important for weight loss. Your body burns more calories even when at rest the more muscle you have. Without the intensity of other workouts, chair yoga helps you tone your body and develop lean muscle. Additionally, stronger muscles can safeguard your joints, which is crucial as you age.

5. Better Digestion: Weight Loss and Nutrient Absorption

A healthy digestive system is supported by yoga. Chair yoga poses and stretches help improve digestion and increase the body's ability to absorb nutrients. When your body receives the proper nutrients, cravings are decreased and healthy eating habits are encouraged.

6. Savor the Flavor When Eating Mindfully

You may include mindful eating into your chair yoga exercise. You may know when you're full and prevent overeating by savoring your food, chewing gently, and being present throughout meals.

7. Getting more rest will help you lose weight quickly.

Sleeping well is a secret to successful weight reduction. Chair yoga promotes healthier sleep patterns, lowers insomnia, and aids in relaxation. A body that has had adequate sleep is better equipped to lose extra weight

Chair yoga is a complete weight-loss strategy that is ideal for women over 40. It is not just about flexibility and relaxation. Your weight reduction journey may be significantly impacted by the mix of mindfulness, light exercise, and overall well being, which will enable you to achieve your objectives with grace and patience.

Nutrition Essentials for Women Over 40

Welcome to the crucial section that will walk you through the dietary components of your chair yoga-based weight reduction journey as a woman over 40. When it comes to maintaining a healthy weight and general wellbeing, this time of life frequently presents particular problems and requirements. I'll discuss how to make sensible, sustainable eating decisions in this chapter as well as the critical role that nutrition plays in your journey toward weight reduction.

Nutritional Balance: The Basis for Weight Loss

Eating properly is just as important for weight reduction as cutting calories. Since our metabolisms tend to slow down as we get older, it's even more important to concentrate on balanced, nutrient-rich diets. A balanced diet helps you maintain a healthy weight and gives you the energy you need for chair yoga.

Foods Rich in Nutrients for Women Over 40

As we become older, it's more crucial than ever to consider the caliber of our meals. Foods that are high in nutrients provide more vitamins, minerals, and antioxidants per calorie, supporting both your general health and weight reduction objectives. Following are some important nutrients and the foods that contain them:

Choose dairy products, leafy greens, and fortified meals to get your daily dose of calcium, which is crucial for maintaining bone health.

Protein: Supports the preservation of muscle mass and might make you feel satisfied for longer. Choose lean sources including tofu, beans, fish, and poultry.

Fiber: Encourages a sense of fullness and aids with digestion. Excellent sources include whole grains, fruits, vegetables, and legumes.

Omega-3 Fatty Acids: Helpful for lowering inflammation and maintaining heart function. Walnuts, flaxseeds, and fatty fish are excellent sources.

Important for the immune system and calcium absorption is vitamin D. Options include fatty fish, sun exposure, and fortified meals.

Planning meals and monitoring portions

Maintaining a healthy weight requires planning meals that are balanced. Consider these helpful advice for meal preparation:

meal: To keep you energized throughout the morning, start your day with a balanced meal that includes protein, fiber, and healthy fats.

Lunch and dinner should include a lot of vegetables, lean meats, and nutritious grains. Beware of excessive quantities.

Snacking: Choose healthy options like Greek yogurt, fruit, almonds, or a handful of raw vegetables.

Hydration: Maintaining a healthy level of hydration is important for general wellbeing and can help stop overeating. The healthiest options for you are water, herbal teas, and infusions.

Controlling portions and eating mindfully

When we reach the age of 40, our eating habits may have changed over time, therefore it's critical to reexamine and engage in mindful eating:

appreciate Every meal: Take your time to appreciate each meal, and chew it completely. This provides your body enough time to detect fullness.

Use Tinier Plates: Using smaller plates and bowls might assist in regulating portion sizes and reducing overeating.

Take Note of Your Body: Pay attention to the signs of hunger and fullness. Eat just when you are hungry, and only when you are full.

Recognize the distinction between actual hunger and emotional eating triggers to avoid emotional eating. Look for different coping mechanisms for stress or emotions.

Weight Loss and Hydration

Drinking enough water is important to remember when trying to lose weight. Maintaining proper hydration can assist your metabolism and aid with appetite management. Here are a few useful tips for staying hydrated:

Every meal should be followed by a glass of water, so make this a habit.

Slices of lemon, cucumber, or berries can be added to infused water to give it a pleasant touch.

Herbal drinks: Herbal teas, including chamomile or green tea, are not only hydrating but also beneficial to your health.

Keep in mind that losing weight is a lengthy process, and that making little, lasting modifications to your diet may have a big impact. You may improve the efficacy of your chair yoga practice and support your weight reduction objectives by concentrating on nutrient-rich meals, portion management, mindful eating, and appropriate hydration.

Combining Yoga with a Balanced Diet

The importance of exercise cannot be overstated in our quest to discover chair yoga's potential as a potent weight-loss strategy for women over 40. What we put on our plates is the other essential element. We'll explore how yoga and a healthy diet may work in harmony to speed and sustain weight reduction in this chapter. We'll talk about how eating right complements the advantages of chair yoga, and we'll offer helpful suggestions for attaining your weight reduction objectives.

The Influence of Balanced Diet on Chair Yoga

As a mild yet effective exercise that improves flexibility, balance, and awareness, chair yoga is perfect for anyone with physical limitations or who are over 40. However, when combined with a healthy diet, its efficiency is greatly increased. This is why:

Understanding a Balanced Diet, Section 1

A balanced diet gives your body the proper nutrients in the appropriate amounts. To make sure you obtain the vital vitamins, minerals, and macronutrients your body requires, it consists of a range of meals from several dietary categories.

1.1 Food Groups and the Role They Play

Fruits and vegetables are excellent providers of dietary fiber, vitamins, and minerals. Find out which are most advantageous for women over 40.

Proteins: Essential for maintaining and repairing muscle. Examine sources of lean protein and portion management.

The body's main source of energy is carbohydrates. Learn the distinction between complex and simple carbohydrates.

1.2 Mindful Eating and Portion Control

The Importance of Portion Control: Recognize proper portion proportions to prevent overeating.

Develop attentive eating habits to avoid emotional or excessive eating when you are eating.

Section 2: Modifying Your Diet for Weight Loss and Chair Yoga

It's necessary to comprehend the fundamentals of a balanced diet, but it's also important to apply these concepts to your chair yoga program and weight reduction objectives.

2.1 Nutrition Prior to and Following Exercise

Choosing pre-workout foods that will provide you prolonged energy will help you get the most out of your chair yoga practice.

The best things to eat after chair yoga for muscle rehabilitation.

2.2 Hydration and Loss of Weight

The Function of Water in Weight reduction: Learn why maintaining hydration is essential to a successful weight reduction plan.

Practical advice to help you fulfill your daily hydration needs are provided in these innovative ways to drink more water.

Section 3: Meal Preparation for Loss of Weight

Planning your meals intentionally can assist you in selecting healthier foods, managing portion sizes, and eventually achieving your weight reduction objectives.

Making a Balanced Meal Plan, Section 3.1

Creating a Daily Meal Plan: A chair yoga-compatible meal plan for ladies over 40.
Timing and Routine of Meals: Recognize the significance of meal frequency and timing for weight reduction.
3.2 Nutritious Snack Selections

Discover wholesome and tasty snack alternatives that won't impede your efforts to lose weight by using smart snacking strategies.

A Lifelong Nutrition and Chair Yoga Approach

Remember that this journey is about more than simply reducing weight as you combine the advantages of chair yoga with a healthy diet. It's about promoting an improved way of life that you can keep up over time. By making the correct food selections, eating slowly, and adjusting your diet to your chair yoga practice, you may lose weight and experience an improvement in your general well-being.

Chapter 5: Yoga for Mindful Eating

Mindfulness and Its Role in Weight Management

It's simple to slip into the trap of mindless eating in today's fast-paced society. Weight gain can be caused by hurried meals, emotional eating, and a lack of awareness.

But do not worry; mindfulness may be your hidden weapon in the fight against obesity. We'll explore how mindfulness may be a key component of weight control in this chapter, particularly when paired with chair yoga for women over 40. A crucial aspect of mindfulness is mindful eating, which may change your relationship with food and aid in weight loss.

Knowledge of mindfulness

Mindfulness is really about being totally in the present. It involves paying attention to your body, your feelings, and your surroundings without passing judgment. When it comes to eating, being mindful means enjoying every meal, observing your hunger and fullness signs, and making deliberate decisions.

Eating mindfully and losing weight:

Slowing Down and Savoring Your Food: Mindful eating causes you to eat more slowly. You take your time enjoying each piece of food rather than scarfing it down quickly. This not only improves your dining experience but also makes it easier for you to know when you're full, helping you avoid overeating.

Listening to Your Body: Mindful eating promotes attentiveness to the messages that your body sends. It's important to eat when you're actually hungry and to quit when you're satiated. This routine can assist you in overcoming emotional eating and pointless munching.

Breaking habitual behaviors: When we're anxious or bored, many of us have habitual eating behaviors that include grabbing for snacks. By being mindful, you may see these tendencies and make better decisions regarding your answers.

Getting Rid of Emotional Eating: Emotional eating is a major barrier to successful weight loss. You may recognize the emotions that are motivating your eating choices and create healthy coping mechanisms with the aid of mindfulness.

meal Control: Mindful eating improves your ability to judge meal sizes. You'll develop the ability to feed yourself the ideal serving size, cutting back on calories.

Chair yoga and mindfulness meditation:

For women over 40, chair yoga is an excellent addition to mindful eating. It encourages relaxation, emotional stability, and bodily awareness. The following is how you may combine these two methods:

Exercise some mindful chair yoga to calm your mind and body before a meal. Put all tension and distractions aside and concentrate only on your breathing. This gets you ready for mindful eating.

Post-Meal Chair Yoga: To promote digestion after a meal, do chair yoga poses. Your body may metabolize food more quickly by using little twists and gentle motions.

Stress management: Chair yoga can be an effective method for controlling stress and emotional eating triggers. You're less likely to resort to food for solace if you lower your stress levels.

Include attentive breathing exercises in your chair yoga program. Making better eating decisions and staying grounded are both facilitated by breath awareness.

Chair yoga and mindfulness may completely change your approach to weight loss. It gives you the power to eat mindfully, make better decisions, and handle your emotions more effectively. By incorporating mindfulness into your everyday life, you'll find it simpler to lose those excess pounds and keep your weight in check. So let's take a deep breath in the present now and enjoy the trip to a better self.

Mindful Eating Strategies

We cannot undervalue the significant impact that mindful eating has on our quest for effective weight loss with chair yoga. The concept of mindful eating encompasses both what you eat and how you eat. It nudges us toward mindful eating, being completely present in the moment, and savoring each meal. Mastering mindful eating can be a game-changer for women over 40 who want to lose those extra pounds. We'll discuss mindful eating in this chapter and how to apply it to your chair yoga for weight reduction journey.

Learning About Mindful Eating

Being completely aware of your dining experience is key to mindful eating. It goes further than calorie tracking and rigid diets. Let's take a closer look:

Pay attention to your body's signals of hunger and fullness by tuning into it. Consume food just when you are actually hungry, not out of habit or boredom.

Use All Your Senses: Investigate the texture, flavor, and scent of your meal using all of your senses. Take note of how wonderful each mouthful is and how it feels in your mouth.

Eat more slowly to give your brain time to catch up with your stomach. Between bites, put your fork down and fully chew your food.

Avoid Distractions: Put away your phone, turn off the TV, and eat at the table. By doing this, you may reduce mindless eating and concentrate on your food.

Controlling portions and eating mindfully

Portion management is aided by mindful eating. Here's how to go about doing it:

Use Smaller Plates: To naturally reduce portion sizes, use smaller plates and bowls.

Instead of setting up serving utensils on the table, serve meals straight from the kitchen. This extra effort may reduce the desire for seconds.

Pay attention to when you feel full, not stuffed, and listen to your body. Your body takes some time to express fullness.

Emotional eating and mindful eating

Emotional eating is a problem for many women. You can handle these emotions with the aid of mindful eating:

Identify Triggers: Recognize the factors that lead to emotional eating. Is it anxiety, boredom, or specific circumstances? The first step to control is awareness.

When you sense the temptation to emotionally eat, pause mindfully. Take many long breaths. Consider if you are indeed hungry or whether another emotional need needs to be met.

Choices in Food and Mindful Eating

The appropriate meal selection is essential for mindful eating:

Choose foods high in nutrients, such as fruits, vegetables, lean meats, and whole grains. Concentrate on Nutrient-Dense Foods.

Make a list of everything you need to buy and follow it. Be careful not to buy unhealthy food on impulse.

Treats are OK, but they should be eaten responsibly. Rather than aimlessly gobbling an entire bar, savor that one piece of chocolate.

Chair yoga while eating mindfully

Chair yoga is an effective method for developing mindful eating:

Yoga before Meals: Before a meal, start with a little chair yoga session. It helps you become more in tune with your body and fosters mindful eating.

Deep breathing exercises might help you stay centered and present while you're eating.

Expressing thankfulness for the food on your plate is a sign of awareness. Recognize the time, energy, and love that went into making it.

By including mindful eating into your chair yoga weight loss journey, you'll be better able to enjoy your meals, make healthier food selections, and control emotional eating. Your relationship to what is on your plate matters more than simply what is on it. You'll find happiness and fulfillment in your meals while attaining your weight reduction objectives if you take the time to enjoy every mouthful.

Chair Yoga for Stress Reduction

Welcome to the chapter on Chair Yoga for Stress Reduction, written especially for women over 40 and a crucial step on your path to mindful eating and weight reduction. Stress may frequently stand in the way of wellbeing in our fast-paced environment. However, you may take advantage of chair yoga's ability to lower stress, improve mindfulness, and assist your weight reduction objectives by including it into your routine. We'll examine how chair yoga may improve your mental and physical balance in this chapter, opening the door to mindful eating and effective weight reduction.

Understanding the Effects of Stress on Weight Loss

All of us are impacted by stress, and for many women over 40, it may be a daily companion. Understanding how stress affects your body and your capacity to keep a healthy weight is essential. Here are some ways that stress might obstruct your efforts to lose weight:

Weight Gain and Stress Hormones: When we are under stress, our bodies release cortisol, sometimes known as the "stress hormone." It might be challenging to maintain a healthy diet when cortisol increases hunger and desires for high-calorie, harmful meals.

Emotional Eating: Stress frequently leads to emotional eating, which makes us go for comfort foods as a means of coping. These emotional eating sessions might result in overeating, which eventually helps people acquire weight.

Reduced Metabolism: Prolonged stress may cause your metabolism to slow down, making it harder to burn calories effectively.

Stress can cause sleep disturbances, and lack of sleep is associated with weight growth. It could make people choose unhealthy foods and not have the energy to exercise.

Chair yoga as a tool for stress reduction

Let's explore how chair yoga may be your stress-reduction ally now:

Chair yoga places a strong emphasis on the relationship between breath and movement. You may quiet your nervous system, lessen tension, and restore control over your emotions with easy breathing exercises and moderate chair positions.

Chair yoga promotes mindfulness by encouraging awareness of the body and its sensations. You may separate yourself from anxious thoughts and discover inner calm by keeping your attention in the here and now.

Improved Sleep: Regular chair yoga practice can improve your sleep quality and stop the stress-related cycle of sleep disruptions. You'll have more energy for your weight reduction journey if you get better sleep.

Explore these chair yoga positions for stress relief to help you relax and release tension. You may relax and reenergize by performing poses like "Seated Forward Bend" and "Chair Cat-Cow".

Chair yoga: Including It in Your Routine

Here's how to include chair yoga into your daily life to reduce stress:

Time Commitment: Set aside a short period of time each day to practice chair yoga. It's a financial investment in your health and your weight-loss objectives.

Find a Quiet, Comfortable Space to Practice Chair Yoga to Create a Relaxing Environment. For increased comfort, use blankets and pillows.

Chair yoga is a mindful eating connection that can help you unwind before meals and encourage mindful eating. Overeating brought on by stress may be avoided by mindful, intentional eating.

Keep Being Consistent: Consistency is essential. You'll notice a favorable effect on your stress levels and, as a result, your weight loss journey as you commit to chair yoga for stress reduction.

Keep in mind that your chair yoga practice is an individual experience. Progress rather than perfection is the goal. You'll be better prepared to make conscious eating choices, support your weight reduction goals, and live a healthier, happier life by lowering stress with chair yoga. Take a deep breath, get into a comfortable chair, and let's start along this stress-free, mindful route to weight reduction.

Chapter 6: Setting Realistic Weight Loss Goals

The Importance of Realistic Goals

Setting realistic objectives must be addressed before we go into the practical components of chair yoga and its tremendous advantages for women over 40 on their weight reduction journey. In this chapter, I'll look at why setting realistic goals is crucial if you want to become a better, happier version of yourself. We'll further divide it into the following subsections:

The Influence of Realism

The compass that directs your weight reduction journey is a set of realistic goals. They help you stay grounded and concentrated on your goals. This idea is more crucial than ever when it comes to chair yoga and losing those excess pounds.

Life occurs, let's face it. Everybody has obligations, commitments, and times when they could stray from their weight-loss goals. Realistic objectives recognize and accommodate this reality. They don't set you up for failure by expecting you to make radical, irreversible changes. Instead, they advocate for slow, steady advancement. Your loyal friend during this journey might be chair yoga mixed with realistic goals.

2. Being aware of your starting point

Recognize where you are right now to start. It's a crucial stage that's frequently skipped, yet realistic goal-setting is built on it. You may choose a beginning point that is compatible with your skills by having a clear awareness of your existing health, fitness level, and daily routine. It doesn't matter if you've practiced chair yoga before or not; what matters is your particular circumstance. Your starting place is unique, and your objectives should be consistent with that.

3. The Function of Persistence and Patience

Both cities and a healthy body take time to develop. It is possible to lose weight gently and sustainably by practicing chair yoga. You are given the gift of patience by setting realistic goals. They are aware that success depends on making constant effort over time. There's no need to expedite the procedure. Rushing really frequently results in exhaustion and disappointment. Allow chair yoga to be your constant companion, and use your goals as a guide to help you improve yourself little by little.

4. Honoring Minor Successes

Your weight reduction journey can be hard, just like life can be. However, if your goals are reasonable, you'll be able to enjoy tiny successes along the road. Every accomplishment, no matter how little, shows your commitment. Even if the goal is still in the distance, these minor victories serve as a source of inspiration and motivation by serving as a reminder that you are making progress on your path.

5. Modifying and Reevaluating

The process of losing weight is also subject to change. Realistic objectives change as your situation does. Realign your goals to reflect your new reality if you encounter setbacks. If your first goals are exceeded, don't be scared to set higher standards. Your route will always be feasible and relevant thanks to this flexibility.

Your allies in the chair yoga for weight reduction path are reasonable goals. They respect your starting point, provide tolerance and support, rejoice in your advancement, and adjust to your changing demands. You'll find that success is not only achievable but also within your reach if you use these objectives as your guide.

I will provide you with guidance in creating these achievable objectives and utilizing chair yoga as a tool to assist you in achieving them in the chapters that follow. Self-compassion and doable steps are the first steps on your path.

Tracking Your Progress and Celebrating Success

Congratulations on starting your chair yoga for weight reduction adventure! Realistic goal-setting is only the first step; monitoring your development is also crucial. I'll go into great detail in this chapter on how to successfully track your accomplishments and, most importantly, how to celebrate them.

Let's face it: losing weight improves your whole health and wellbeing, not just the numbers on the scale. This chapter will walk you through useful techniques for evaluating your development and appreciating the good changes taking place inside of you.

Beginning with Baseline Measurements in Sub-Section 1

Establishing a starting point is essential before talking about measuring development. You need a starting point to compare your accomplishments to. What you can do is:

Weight: First, weigh yourself and record the result. Consider weekly or monthly trends rather than daily figures because your weight might vary regularly.

Take measures of your waist, hips, and thighs, as well as other important body parts. When it comes to changes in body composition, these metrics may be more insightful than simply weight.

Before-and-After Pictures: Think about capturing "before" pictures from various perspectives. These images can provide compelling visual proof of your development.

Keeping a Weight Loss Journal in Sub-Section 2

A weight loss notebook serves as your own journey log. You can keep track of the following in a notepad, specialized program, or easy spreadsheet:

Daily Food Intake: Keep track of your meals and beverages. This will enable you to see trends and choose your diet with knowledge.

Physical activity: Keep a journal of your chair yoga sessions, including how you felt and any adjustments you made. Yoga progress tracking is a great approach to see changes over time.

Mood and Energy Levels: Keep track of your day-to-day mental health and energy levels. This might show the effects that lifestyle modifications are having on your general health.

Setting Realistic Milestones in Sub-Section 3

Setting realistic goals is essential for keeping motivation high and monitoring development. Remember the following advice:

Short-Term Goals: Divide your long-term objective into more manageable, time-bound goals. For instance, try to improve your ability to do a certain chair yoga posture or strive to lose two to three pounds in a month.

Celebrate your non-scale accomplishments, such as greater flexibility, more endurance, or better sleep. These are equally significant to the scale's numbers.

Regular Progress Assessments: Subsection 4

Regular yet non-obsessive progress evaluation is crucial. This is how:

Weigh-In Routine: Weigh yourself once a week or once a month at the same time and under identical circumstances, for as just after using the restroom in the morning.

Measure your body again every couple of weeks to observe how your body is evolving.

Compare your "before" and "after" images on a regular basis to visually track your physical changes.

Subsection 5: Honoring Achievement

The trip is made up in large part of celebrating your victories. It helps you recognize the effort you are putting in and keeps you motivated:

Reward Yourself: When you reach a goal, reward yourself with something enjoyable that won't impede your growth. A movie night, a spa day, or a new book may be on the agenda.

Don't be afraid to brag about your accomplishments to your friends or in a group that is encouraging. Positive reinforcement from others may be a strong motivator.

Remind yourself of your successes and the constructive adjustments you've made. Recognize your work and be kind to yourself.

Progress monitoring and achievement celebration are continuous processes. It's about realizing that every step you take toward greater health and fitness, no matter how tiny, counts as progress. Therefore, enjoy each success, no matter how small, and continue working toward your goals. You can do this.

Staying Motivated on Your Weight Loss Journey

Starting a weight reduction journey is similar to embarking on a brand-new voyage. Your dedication is first fueled by early excitement, but as you travel through the ups and downs of your journey, your resolve may falter. Through the perspective of Chair Yoga for Women Over 40, we'll explore the crucial subject of keeping motivated on your weight reduction journey in this chapter.

Setting attainable weight loss objectives

Why Realistic Goals Are Important

Setting realistic weight reduction goals is essential for getting your motivation going and keeping it going. Why? Because you may achieve success by using attainable goals as stepping stones. They help you maintain your sense of purpose and keep you from feeling overburdened. Your objectives transform from targets into motivating milestones when they are in line with your talents.

Recognizing SMART Goals

Using SMART objectives is one tried-and-true technique for establishing these milestones:

Specific: Clearly state the goals you have in mind. For instance, "I want to lose 10 pounds" is more precise than "I want to lose weight."
Measurable: To monitor your advancement, take precise measurements. "I will track my weight every week" is a quantifiable technique to measure your success.
Achievable: Make sure your objectives are doable. For some people, but not all, aiming to drop 10 pounds in a month may be reasonable. Make the goal feasible.

Relevant: Your objectives have to be in line with your diet strategy. Relevant objectives for chair yoga practitioners can include increasing flexibility or strengthening certain muscle areas.

Time-bound: Give your objectives a time period. Adding the phrase "I will lose 10 pounds in three months" creates a sense of urgency.

Process of Setting Goals

Set long-term objectives first: What is your long-term weight loss objective? Make a note of it and picture it.

Take it apart: Break up your long-term objective into smaller, more doable short-term objectives. Set a goal of losing two to three pounds every month, for instance, if your goal is to lose 20 pounds in six months.

Review and reevaluate frequently: Reevaluate your progress frequently, and change your goals as necessary.

It's acceptable to change your goals as required because life does happen.
Avoiding Common Mistakes

Making Comparisons to Others: Your experience is special to you. Comparing your development to that of another person can be demoralizing. Aim to follow your own path.
Strive for progress rather than perfection. Since nobody is flawless, mistakes happen frequently. Take care of yourself.
Setting unreasonable goals: Losing weight should be sustained and progressive. Setting objectives that are too ambitious might result in fatigue and disappointment.
Monitoring Progress

It's essential to monitor your development if you want to stay motivated. Think about keeping a notebook where you may keep track of your chair yoga sessions, dietary adjustments, and any weight reduction successes. A powerful motivator, progress monitoring gives you a visual depiction of your progress.

In a nutshell, SMART objectives should direct the road toward weight loss and wellbeing. These objectives make sure that no matter the difficulties, you remain motivated and committed to your journey. Remember that your journey is individual, be gentle to yourself, and practice mindfulness. Your weight reduction goals will be easier to reach and your motivation will remain strong if you follow these guidelines.

Chapter 7: Chair Yoga Challenges and Solutions

Addressing Common Challenges Faced by Women Over 40

Life may be a lovely adventure, but when women approach the age of 40, they frequently encounter particular difficulties with regard to their health, fitness, and weight control. It's crucial to be aware of these difficulties and, more significantly, to come up with workable answers. I'll explore the typical obstacles older women encounter while trying to lose weight using chair yoga in this chapter. I'll provide you insightful tips, useful counsel, and successful methods to get beyond these obstacles and accomplish your objectives.

Part 1: Physical Difficulties

Age-Related Pain and Stiffness

Age-related stiffness and joint pain are among the most prevalent physical difficulties experienced by women over 40. Yoga in a chair is a fantastic remedy for this. It eases your body into stretches gradually, increasing flexibility and minimizing pain.

Solutions:

Start with easy chair yoga postures that concentrate on your trouble spots.

Your chair yoga practices should be gradually extended in order to develop strength and flexibility.

Use props to support your body and ease into positions, such as pillows and cushions.

Metabolism Slowdown

As we become older, our metabolism slows down, making it harder to lose those extra pounds. Your metabolism may be reactivated with chair yoga, which can help you lose weight.

Solutions:

Include energizing, flowing chair yoga sequences to increase your metabolism and heart rate.

Chair yoga should be practiced in conjunction with a nutritious diet to promote a healthy metabolic rate.

Section 2: Inspirational Obstacles

Limited time

There may not be much time for exercise when juggling job, family, and other obligations. A useful solution that enables you to exercise even in little periods of time is chair yoga.

Solutions:

Plan brief chair yoga breaks throughout the day, either before bed or during work breaks.
Include chair yoga in your regular practice by stretching gently while watching TV, for example.
Motivational Lows and Stalls

It's disappointing when weight reduction reaches a plateau. It's essential to remain motivated throughout these moments.

Solutions:

Create attainable, realistic goals so you can monitor your progress and stay motivated.
To overcome plateaus, experiment with various chair yoga poses and mix up your routine.
Section 3: Mental Health Issues

Self-Esteem and Body Image

Our bodies alter as we age. It's typical to battle with one's self-esteem and body image, which makes getting in shape and losing weight much harder.

Solutions:

Adopt a body-positive mindset and develop self-compassion.
Set objectives that focus on bettering your health and wellbeing rather than merely your beauty.
Emotional eating and stress

Stress tends to get worse as we age and might trigger emotional eating. Utilizing chair yoga can help you better manage stress and emotional triggers by encouraging relaxation and awareness.

Solutions:

Utilize chair yoga's mindfulness and deep breathing methods to alleviate stress.

To treat emotional eating tendencies, ask friends, family, or specialists for assistance.
Conclusion

Age is simply a number, and women over 40 may overcome the obstacles to weight reduction they confront by being persistent, having patience, and using the correct resources. Chair yoga is a holistic method of well-being that tackles both physical and psychological difficulties. It is more than just a workout program. On the other hand, you'll find a healthier, happier version of yourself if you accept these answers and remain dedicated to your quest.

Modifications for Physical Limitations

I'm aware that not everyone begins their chair yoga for weight reduction journey from the same physical condition. Each of us has a special body with physical limits. These difficulties, such as joint discomfort, stiffness, or movement issues, might make yoga appear scary. But do not worry; chair yoga is here to offer a remedy. This chapter will explore the many physical restrictions you could have and provide helpful tips for overcoming them. No matter where you're beginning from, we think chair yoga may be beneficial.

1. Joint discomfort and stiffness

Joint pain and stiffness may be a daily struggle for many women over 40. Due to these problems, conventional yoga positions may be unpleasant or difficult. However, chair yoga offers a fantastic substitute. For stiffness and joint discomfort, alter as follows:

To ease the load on your joints, substitute sitting variations for standing ones.
Gentle motions: To prevent unexpected shocks to your joints, make gentle, controlled motions.
During postures, use cushions or blocks to support your joints and increase comfort.
Insufficient Mobility:

Chair yoga may be your greatest buddy if you have trouble moving about. These adjustments are made to ensure your comfort while moving around:

Exercises that operate inside your comfortable range of motion should be your main priority.

Choose sitting twists to increase the flexibility and mobility of your spine.

Holding onto a chair might help you maintain your balance and stability when performing standing positions.

3. Backache:

Back discomfort is a frequent problem, so it's important to treat it gently while doing chair yoga. These changes can be beneficial:

Back Support: To keep your spine aligned, sit on a chair with the right back support.
Gently bend your back, concentrating on flexibility rather than excessive bending.
Deep breathing can help to relieve back muscular tension, so practice mindful breathing.
4. Balance Issues

Being balanced may be difficult, especially as we become older. You may increase your stability when doing chair yoga:

One-Legged Pose: To start, practice one-legged positions while holding a chair for balance.

Pay great attention to the transitions between positions to avoid falling.

Work on strengthening your core to improve overall stability.

5. Chronic Illnesses:

Chair yoga may be customized to meet the requirements of women who are managing chronic health conditions:

If you have a chronic ailment, always get the advice of your healthcare physician before beginning a yoga practice.

Adjust as Required: Adapt your postures and motions to your condition's needs.
Emphasize pain-free mobility and abstain from excessive activity.

Your physical restrictions shouldn't stop you from taking advantage of chair yoga's amazing weight-loss advantages. With these adjustments, you may adapt chair yoga to your particular needs while incorporating it into your practice safely and successfully. Keep in mind that chair yoga is here to help you along the way at every stage of your journey.

Finding Support and Community

Starting a chair yoga weight reduction journey may be a rewarding and life-changing event. You don't have to do it alone, though, so keep that in mind. Your success can depend on the backing of a group of people who share your values. We'll go into the crucial role that community and finding support play in conquering the difficulties of chair yoga for women over 40 and weight reduction in this chapter.

Why Community and Support Are Important

merely does losing weight involve losing weight, but it also involves converting to a healthy lifestyle. This path may be made more doable, fun, and sustainable with the help of a community. Here is why it's important:

Accountability: You are more likely to stick to your practice and weight reduction plan when you have a group of friends or other yoga practitioners who share your goals.

Motivation: Observing others who are doing similar journeys succeed or get over challenges may be a strong motivator. It serves as a reminder that you can achieve your goals.

Knowledge Exchange: A community is a great location to pick up tips from others. You may learn fresh chair yoga techniques, effective strategies for losing weight, and dietary secrets.

Support on an Emotional Level: Losing weight is a journey on both an emotional and a physical level. A caring group of people may offer inspiration, compassion, and a secure setting in which to discuss successes and setbacks.

How to Find Community and Support

Now that you know why community and support are important, let's look at where to locate these components for your chair yoga and weight-loss journey:

Look for chair yoga sessions in your neighborhood. Attend a few to meet others who share your interests and objectives. You may create in-person friendships by enrolling in local classes.

Online Communities: There are several forums, social media pages, and websites on the internet that are devoted to chair yoga and weight reduction for women over 40. Join these online forums to exchange stories, pose inquiries, and find inspiration.

Find an accountability partner or a fitness companion who will participate with you in chair yoga sessions and weight reduction efforts. You may share your advancement and keep each other inspired.

On social media sites like Instagram and YouTube, follow yoga teachers, dietitians, and fitness professionals. Numerous them provide daily motivation, chair yoga exercises, and tips for leading healthy lives.

Creating Your Own Support System

Consider founding your own community if you can't locate the suitable one. This is how:

Host Chair Yoga Sessions: Host chair yoga sessions in your house with friends or family. You can alternate leading, exchange wholesome treats, and support one another.

Create a Social Media Group: With friends or like-minded people who are interested in chair yoga and weight reduction, start a private social media group. Exchange stories and advice with one another.

Attend seminars and retreats: Look for chair yoga retreats or programs that are tailored to women over 40. These gatherings frequently help you make contacts with other attendees who have similar objectives.

Inference: You Are Not Alone

Finding community and support is a crucial component of chair yoga and weight loss for women over 40. You may get the extra push you require to accomplish your objectives from the friends you make, the inspiration you receive, and the information you pick up from others. Keep in mind that many people are willing to accompany you on your trip and that you are not alone in it. Through chair yoga and weight reduction, you may encourage, boost, and support one another as you embrace a better, happier life.

Chapter 8: Staying Active and Engaged

Incorporating Chair Yoga into Your Daily Routine

Welcome to a crucial phase of your chair yoga journey to remaining active and involved! In this chapter, we'll look at how to include chair yoga into your daily routine so that you can keep up a regular practice that supports your weight reduction objectives. Whether you're new to chair yoga or have some expertise, we'll offer helpful tips for incorporating it successfully into your daily routine.

A Morning Routine for Chair Yoga to Start Your Day

By including chair yoga in your morning practice, you may start the day off feeling rejuvenated. This is how:

The day should begin with a gentle awakening and the establishing of good thoughts. Locate a cozy chair in a peaceful area.

Deep breathing exercises should be done in the morning to awaken your body and mind. Exhale gently through your lips while taking a slow, deep breath through your nose to relax.

Practice a modified version of the traditional yoga Sun Salutation routine while seated. These easy stretches strengthen your body and increase flexibility.

Adding Chair Yoga to Your Lunch Break to Revitalize Your Afternoons

A noon energy boost may be achieved with your chair yoga exercise. To start, try these:

Desk yoga stretches: If you spend your days at a desk, take a few minutes to practice chair yoga. To reduce stress, try shoulder rolls, sitting twists, and wrist stretches.

Deep Breathing for Stress Reduction: Take a few slow, deep breaths to fight the afternoon slump. Repeat numerous times, inhaling for four counts, holding for four, and exhaling for four.

Set aside 10 to 15 minutes for a brief chair yoga session. Concentrate on forward bends in the sitting position and side stretches to increase blood flow and improve focus.

Evening Chair Yoga to De-Stress and Prepare for Sleep

Chair yoga can help you unwind as your day comes to a close and get ready for a good night's sleep. Think about these techniques:

Wind-Down Poses: To relieve any tension that has built up, wind down with easy stretches like neck rolls, shoulder releases, and sitting spinal twists.

Spend a few minutes in sitting meditation to practice mindfulness. Bring your focus to the current moment and concentrate on your breathing. It can enhance sleep quality and lessen stress.

Breathing for Sleep: Use relaxation techniques, such as the 4-7-8 breathing technique, to create the calmness necessary for sleep. Breathe in for four counts, hold for seven, and then let out for eight.

Weekly Chair Yoga Challenges: A Enjoyable and Diverse Program

Consider these weekly challenges to keep your chair yoga practice interesting:

Chair yoga poses for balance and core development should be practiced on one day each week. Try modified boat posture, knee extensions, and sitting leg lifts.

Select a day for longer stretches and relaxation as your "flexibility and relaxation day." Include postures like the butterfly stretch, sitting pigeon, and chair yoga.

Finish each practice session with an expression of thanks. Consider your accomplishments, journey, and how chair yoga is helping you attain your weight reduction objectives.

You're investing in your health by including chair yoga into your everyday routine. This routine fosters emotional harmony and mental clarity in addition to improving your physical health. Keep in mind that repetition is the key, so be dedicated and have fun as you progress with chair yoga. It's a crucial tool for helping you lose weight and keeps you interested and active as you age gracefully.

Let's put these concepts into action now and design a chair yoga program for daily use that suits you.

Making Physical Activity a Habit

Congratulations on starting your chair yoga weight reduction journey! This chapter will go into detail on how important it is to incorporate regular physical activity into your everyday routine. We are aware that life may be hectic and that finding time to work out is not always simple. However, you'll discover the secret to long-lasting health and vigor by developing the chair yoga habit.

The Secret to Long-Term Success Is Forming a Habit

Any new effort may be thrilling and inspiring to begin, such as chair yoga for weight reduction. However, genuine change only occurs with constancy. You're more likely to persist with exercise over the long term if you make it a habit.

Knowledge of Habit Formation

It's helpful to comprehend the science of habit formation. Your brain automatically repeats acts that have become habits without your conscious awareness. Forming a new habit requires effort and repetition over time. This is how you do it:

1. Start Modestly:

Start with attainable targets. Commit, for instance, to daily chair yoga for 10 minutes. This makes it less intimidating, which increases your chances of success.
2. Maintaining Consistency:

Set aside a definite time and location to practice chair yoga. Consistency makes it easier for your brain to identify and integrate the habit into your everyday routine.

3. Employ triggers

Connect your chair yoga routine to an established routine, such as drinking your morning tea or watching your preferred TV program. You can be reminded to exercise by this trigger.

4. Give Yourself a Treat:

Your chair yoga practices deserve some modest treats. The habit is strengthened by these advantageous associations. It may be as easy as unwinding with a cup of herbal tea afterwards.

Overcoming Typical Obstacles

The process of forming habits isn't always easy. Here are some typical issues and workable solutions:

1. Time Restrictions:

We all have busy schedules. Consider breaking up your chair yoga practice into smaller sessions throughout the day to get around this.
2. Insufficient Motivation

Start with a vow to yourself to practice for only a few minutes on days when you're lacking motivation. Once you get started, you'll frequently notice that your motivation rises.

Third, boredom

Change up your routine if chair yoga gets stale. To keep it interesting, experiment with different positions, watch instructional chair yoga videos, or make your own mix of calming music.

4. Responsibility

Inform a friend or relative of your dedication to chair yoga. They could encourage you and support you, which would make skipping your practice more difficult.

Keeping a Journal: Its Power

For habit building, keeping a chair yoga notebook can be a game-changer. Keep track of your daily practice, your feelings while doing it, and any advancements you see. Writing in a journal gives you a sense of success and inspires you to keep going on your quest.

Like chair yoga, developing a fitness routine involves integrating it into your daily routine. The routine becomes automatic once you accept it. Always keep in mind that tiny, persistent efforts over time produce big results. Maintain your motivation and allow chair yoga to become a fun and necessary aspect of your everyday life.

Staying Socially Connected

In order to be active and involved while doing chair yoga to lose weight, maintaining social relationships is crucial. This chapter will examine the significant benefits of maintaining social connections and how they might improve your practice of chair yoga. Additionally, we'll discuss straightforward, doable methods for growing and maintaining your social network.

The Influence of Social Interaction

The value of maintaining social connections as we become older becomes more and more clear. Social connection has a significant impact on our general wellbeing and the effectiveness of our weight reduction efforts. It is not simply about providing company. Let's see how everything functions.

The Importance of Social Connection
There are many advantages to connecting with others, whether it is in a chair yoga session or on a group stroll. Here is why it's important:

Mental and Emotional Well-Being: Participating in a chair yoga session alongside friends and peers develops a sense of belonging, which lowers feelings of isolation and despair. Maintaining motivation and commitment to your weight reduction objectives requires a positive outlook.

Accountability and Support: Having a network of accountability is created by sharing your story with others. Your yoga partners can motivate you to attend sessions frequently, try out new positions, and maintain your attention on your weight reduction goals.

Social learning: Chair yoga classes provide a forum for discussing observations and experiences. Through applying their methods to your own path, you can gain knowledge from other people's achievements and failures.

Inspiration and Motivation: Observing other participants' progress can inspire and motivate you. It serves as a reminder that reaching your goals is possible, regardless of your age.

Practical Advice for Remaining Socially Active:

1. Attend Yoga Classes Nearby:

Find chair yoga lessons near you. These sessions provide you the chance to connect with people who share your interests and are like-minded.
Join in on group activities before or after class, such meet-ups for tea or coffee, to foster relationships.
2. Communities for Yoga Online:

Examine social media groups for women over 40 and online chair yoga forums.

Join a community of like-minded individuals, exchange ideas, and discuss your progress. Virtual assistance is easily accessible and advantageous.

3. Participate in seminars and workshops:

Visit health fairs, wellness lectures, and chair yoga lessons. These gatherings bring people together who share a passion for wellbeing.

Participate in conversations and socialize with participants.

4. Volunteering and Networking

Participate in community or charitable events as a volunteer. In addition to helping others, volunteering gives you a chance to make new acquaintances.

Creating connections with others who share your beliefs may be a great source of support.

5. Set social objectives

Take on the weekly challenge of striking up a conversation with one new person. These casual interactions have the potential to develop into lifelong friendships.

Conclusion:

Your chair yoga weight reduction journey is not an alone one. Maintaining social connections enhances the process, promotes your wellness objectives, and makes the whole thing more fun. Utilize these useful suggestions to improve your relationships with others and build a vibrant community around your fitness quest.

You'll encourage one another to continue being active, involved, and dedicated to your weight reduction goals.

Chapter 9: Inspirational Stories and Testimonials

Real-Life Success Stories from Women Over 40

Real-life success tales from women over 40 serve as beacons of encouragement in the field of chair yoga and weight loss. These extraordinary ladies have transformed their life by using the power of chair yoga to lose weight and improve their overall health and well-being. Their experiences serve as a reminder that it is never too late to start a better lifestyle. We'll go further into the stories of these remarkable women in this chapter, hearing about their struggles, successes, and the significant effects chair yoga has had on their weight reduction objectives.

Finding Balance and Confidence on Carla's Journey

Carla, a young and active woman in her late 40s, was struggling with extra weight that had gathered over time. Her confidence was eroding as she felt the weight both physically and mentally. Her epiphany was chair yoga. She started out gently and gradually with some fundamental chair yoga positions. Carla gained a new feeling of balance and inner power under her instructor's kind instruction. She began to regard weight reduction as a side effect of her quest for wellbeing rather than the main goal. Her progress in losing weight was a consistent, healthy 1-2 pounds every week. The example of Carla shows us how chair yoga may be a sympathetic companion on our weight reduction quest.

Linda's Victory: Surmounting Mobility Issues

Linda, who was in her early 50s, had experienced movement problems as a result of a medical ailment. She felt stuck in a cycle of weight gain due to her restricted capacity to engage in traditional exercise. It was chair yoga that saved her. She liked how flexible the technique was and used a chair as support. She eventually lost the extra weight and regained her mobility via constant work. Linda's story serves as proof that women with mobility issues may find empowerment in chair yoga.

Gloria's Mind-Body Connection: Weight Loss and Stress Reduction

Gloria, a professional mother of 49, managed a busy life and saw how stress affected her weight. She first learned about the fundamental link between the mind and body through chair yoga. She discovered how to relax with her breath, and she also started doing chair yoga. As her cortisol levels decreased, the weight started to go. Gloria's experience serves as a reminder of the effective stress-reduction and weight-loss effects of chair yoga.

Chair yoga as a way of life for Mary: Her Joyful Transformation

Mary thought it was time for a change at the age of 45. She adopted chair yoga as a way of life rather than merely an activity. She included chair yoga into her daily regimen, including calming positions before bed and gentle morning stretches. She found a consistent road to weight loss with her newly acquired discipline. Mary's tale serves as a reminder of the value of reliability and dedication in chair yoga's function as a lifestyle option for women over 40.

These accounts of Carla, Linda, Gloria, and Mary provide illuminating illustrations of how chair yoga may be an effective weight reduction aid for women over 40. Their personal stories serve as a reminder that chair yoga is about achieving balance, resilience, and a healthier, more vibrant version of oneself, not only about losing weight. Their experiences demonstrate the value of tenacity, flexibility, and self-care in the quest for a healthy way of life. Let these women's inspiration encourage you to begin your journey towards wellness with hope and confidence as we explore the worlds of chair yoga and weight reduction.

How Chair Yoga Transformed Lives

The amazing effects chair yoga has had on the lives of women over 40 are explored in this chapter, along with the motivational tales and testimonies that serve as evidence of its transformational power. We see how chair yoga evolved into more than simply a workout regimen; it became a lifeline, a source of strength, and a catalyst for significant transformation via personal tales and shared experiences.

Regaining Health and Vitality after Mobility Struggles:

Mobility problems and physical limits can be difficult for many women over 40 to get over. Activities that were once routine and simple become difficult. However, the testimonies we've collected demonstrate that chair yoga has been a game-changer, sparking fresh hope and resiliency.

Finding Freedom in Movement: Susan's Story

Susan, who was in her mid-fifties, was dealing with joint discomfort and having restricted mobility. Traditional exercise seemed difficult to contemplate. She felt liberated in a new way because of the support and gentle movements of chair yoga. "Chair yoga gave me the joy of movement back," says Susan. My physique no longer makes me feel confined. Every day is like a celebration of what my body is capable of.

Chair yoga for confidence-building

As her weight rose, Karen, a lady in her late 40s, experienced problems with her self-esteem. She had the chance to rebuild self-assurance via chair yoga. According to her, chair yoga is about learning to appreciate your body and yourself, not just the physical positions. It's a path toward accepting oneself.

Chair yoga and mental well-being can help you embrace peace and manage stress.

Stress is a hidden enemy that frequently becomes worse with age and has a negative impact on both physical and mental health. Chair yoga provides comfort and mental clarity in addition to its physical advantages.

The Peaceful Travels of Emma

Emma, a lady in her 40s, was under a lot of stress at work and in her personal life. She learned mindfulness and relaxation skills via chair yoga. She explains, "It's like a reset button for my mind." "I've discovered how to release tension and concentrate on the here and now. Every day, I treat myself to it as a gift.

Newfound Vitality and Energy

Catherine, who is in her early 50s, attests to the positive effects of chair yoga on her level of energy. "I was often exhausted, but chair yoga gave me energy. It serves as my body's equivalent of a cup of coffee. My day begins with enthusiasm and hope.

Chair yoga as a sustainable weight-loss route to a healthier you

A lot of women over 40 are working toward a healthy weight, and chair yoga is essential to this process. These testimonies show how chair yoga assisted in significant weight reduction breakthroughs.

A Sustainable Change in Lifestyle

Carol, who is in her fifties, stresses the longevity of weight loss with chair yoga. "I wasn't a fan of fad diets or strenuous exercise. I started doing chair yoga every day, and it changed how I felt about eating. Long-term health is important; weight loss is only one aspect of it.
A Lifelong Transformational Journey

The case studies and accounts you've just read serve as tangible evidence of the extraordinary positive effects chair yoga can have on the lives of women over 40. It's more than just a workout regimen; it's a transformational path toward empowerment, stress reduction, and long-term weight loss. The benefits of chair yoga go beyond the physical; they also affect the soul and promote a closer relationship with oneself. We are motivated by the experiences to go out on our own journeys and experience chair yoga's transformative effects.

Chapter 10: Embracing Wellness and Self-Care

Self-Care Rituals for Women Over 40

Welcome to a chapter written just for you—a woman over 40 who needs a bit more tender loving care. We frequently neglect to prioritize ourselves in the midst of life's chaos. But in this chapter, I'll look at self-care practices that are personalized for you, with an emphasis on embracing wellness and self-care as you start your chair yoga for weight loss journey.

Self-Care's Influence on Women Over 40
It's important to comprehend the enormous effects that self-care practices may have on your general well-being before we get into any particular routines, especially for women in their 40s. Here are some reasons why self-care is essential to your journey:

Management of Stress:

Due to obligations to your family, work, and other commitments, your 40s may be a stressful decade. You may improve your mental health and manage stress and anxiety by engaging in self-care routines.
Physical Well-Being:

Self-care supports your weight reduction objectives and promotes healthy aging, chronic illness prevention, and physical well-being.

3. Emotional Fortitude

You could experience emotional difficulties as you mature. Self-care strengthens your emotional resiliency and enables you to gracefully handle life's ups and downs.

4. Individual Empowerment

You can feel empowered and more confident by prioritizing your needs and asserting your value via self-care.

Positive Self-Care Practices

Let's look at some nourishing self-care practices designed especially for ladies over the age of 40:

1. Morning meditation
Spend a few minutes being aware in the morning. Look, choose a calm area, settle in, and concentrate on your breathing. This routine might help you start the day off right and confront problems with a clear head.

2. Chair Yoga to Reduce Stress
Add chair yoga to your everyday schedule. Pick relaxing positions that will help you relax and release tension. Yoga has the power to change your flexibility and stress levels.

3. Taking Care of Your Body
Keep a watchful eye on your diet. Place a focus on nutrient-rich foods that aid in weight loss and general wellness. Include a mix of fruits and vegetables, complete grains, and lean proteins in your meals.

4. **Habit of Hydration**
Make it a habit to drink water. Maintaining energy levels and assisting in weight reduction require proper hydration. Carry a reusable water bottle, and aim to stay hydrated all day long.

5. Nighttime Rest
In the evening, unwind with a soothing routine. To relieve any day's worth of stress that has built up, try a

warm bath, deep breathing exercises, or gentle chair yoga stretches.

6. Relationship with Nature

Spend some time outside. It is peaceful and revitalizing to be in nature. Take a stroll, do some yoga in your garden, or just sit outside and take in the beauty of nature.

7. Restful Sleep

Putting sleep first. Make sure you receive adequate rejuvenating sleep every night. A restful night's sleep is essential for maintaining your physical and mental health.

8. Encourage Originality

Take up creative activities. Whether it's drawing, writing, or playing an instrument, being creative can be a delight and a way to express oneself.

9. Social Assistance

Develop your social networks. Spend time with family and friends to strengthen your feeling of community and your emotional support system.

Final Thoughts

Keep in mind that self-care is a requirement, especially for women over 40. These self-care practices can improve your general wellbeing and work in harmony with your chair yoga practice. You are moving much closer to attaining your wellness and weight reduction objectives by adopting self-care. So go ahead and include self-care into your daily schedule without hesitation. You'll be grateful to your body and mind.

The Holistic Approach to Health and Wellness

It's important to pause and think about our well-being in a society that frequently passes us by, especially for women over 40. The holistic approach is your constant partner in developing and sustaining a healthy and balanced existence. This chapter will go into the idea of holistic wellbeing, examine chair yoga specifically designed for women over 40, and investigate the fundamental relationship between mindfulness and successful weight reduction.

The Building Blocks of Holistic Health

The concept of holistic wellness encompasses the notion that well being includes a harmonic balance between the mind, body, and spirit in addition to the absence of disease. Let's dissect this strategy:

Physical Wellness: Caring for your body via exercise, a healthy diet, and enough sleep include being physically well. Women over 40 should be aware of their natural changes and give their bodies the attention they need to flourish.

Mental and Emotional Wellness: It's important to manage stress, cultivate a good outlook, and promote emotional resilience. Chair yoga has the potential to be a potent technique for improving emotional stability and mental equilibrium.

Spiritual Wellness: Connecting to your inner self, discovering meaning, and finding purpose are all aspects of spirituality, which need not always imply religion. Excellent wellness techniques for this area of wellbeing include chair yoga and mindfulness.

Chair Yoga for Women Over 40: What You Need to Know

Definition of Chair Yoga: Chair yoga is a mild style of yoga that combines several poses and stretches that are all supported by a chair. It's ideal for anyone searching for a low-impact form of exercise or those who may have physical restrictions.

Physical advantages: Maintaining strength, balance, and flexibility become more crucial as women age. These demands are met by chair yoga while harm risk is kept to a minimum.

Chair yoga is a comprehensive practice that incorporates awareness, breathing techniques, and meditation in addition to physical forms. It can aid in lowering stress, improving mental acuity, and fostering emotional wellbeing.

The Role of the Mind and Body in Weight Loss

Knowing the Mind-Body Connection: Your ideas and feelings may significantly affect your physical well-being and weight. For example, stress might result in emotional eating and weight gain. With its focus on mindfulness, chair yoga enables you to become more aware of your body's demands.

Embracing Mindful Eating: One of the things that makes chair yoga so magical is its capacity to foster awareness. You'll discover how to appreciate the flavor of your meal, identify hunger and fullness cues, and select healthier foods.

Stress Reduction and Weight Loss: Emotional eating is less frequent when stress is adequately managed via exercises like chair yoga. Losing stress encourages healthy eating and overall well being.

Chair yoga for women over 40 is a potent technique that addresses both the physical and emotional components of health in the holistic road to wellbeing. It's a conscientious and practical strategy to advance your weight-loss objectives while enhancing your general wellbeing.

Conclusion

Honoring Your Accomplishments

Now that we have reached the end of "Chair Yoga for Women Over 40: Weight Loss," let's take a minute to recognize and congratulate all that you have accomplished. This is an incredible trip that you have started. You've acknowledged the need for change, acted upon it, and enjoyed the benefits of your tenacity and devotion.

Accepting Your Achievements

Realizing that each stride you've made, each chair yoga posture you've perfected, and each mindful moment you've welcomed has all contributed to your journey is crucial. Every accomplishment, regardless of size, is cause for celebration, whether it involves losing weight or just developing a fresh respect for your physical appearance.

Your wellness and health achievements

Maybe you've noticed a difference in your physical well-being: you feel stronger, more nimble, and have more flexibility. Perhaps you've observed an improvement in your mental and emotional health, feeling less anxious, more focused, and more capable of overcoming obstacles in life. Your overall health has improved. This is a positive development.

A Healthy Lifetime

The holistic approach to wellbeing and health is beautiful because it goes much beyond what you'll find in this book. It's a trip that lasts a lifetime, and you have the resources and understanding to carry on with assurance and grace.

Your Ongoing Path to Better Health and Loss of Weight

Your journey is far from done when you flip the last page of this book—in fact, it has only just begun. The following doable actions will guarantee your ongoing success:

1. Set New Objectives: Recognize the value of goal-setting. Whether your goals are to maintain your present weight, lose more weight, or improve your chair yoga practice, setting fresh objectives can help you stay motivated and focused.

2. Remain Consistent: Long-term success requires consistency. Maintain mindful eating practices, go on with your chair yoga practice, and make self-care an indispensable part of your everyday routine.

3. Seek Support: Don't be afraid to get in touch with a support group, a dietician, or a chair yoga teacher. Being surrounded by people who support and understand you on your path may be really helpful.

4. Reflect and Adjust: Continually evaluate your success and make necessary adjustments to your strategy. It's acceptable to make adjustments along the way because the road to weight reduction and wellness is not always straight.

5. Self-Compassion: Take care of yourself first and foremost. Recognize that failures are inevitable and that they are only steps on the path to your ultimate achievement. Proceed on your path with self-compassion and patience.

A healthy lifestyle awaits.

The path to better health and weight loss is a fulfilling one that changes over time rather than ending. You now have a thorough knowledge of chair yoga's ability to change not just your physical state but also your mental and spiritual state. You've made self-care, balance, and mindfulness a priority in your life.

Recall that you are not alone in your journey to health and well-being. You possess the inner fortitude and knowledge necessary to turn this into a lifetime of health. Once ignored, your body and spirit are now your most valued allies. Honor your accomplishments since they serve as the cornerstone for the rest of your trip.

This is the start of a brand-new chapter in your life, not merely the conclusion of a book. The way forward is clear; there are countless options, and you have the ability to control your own fate. It is a path of self-discovery, self-care, and self-love that leads to health and weight loss. Thus, move on with self-assurance and create a masterpiece of wellbeing out of your existence. Your bright future, full of energy and health, is waiting for you.

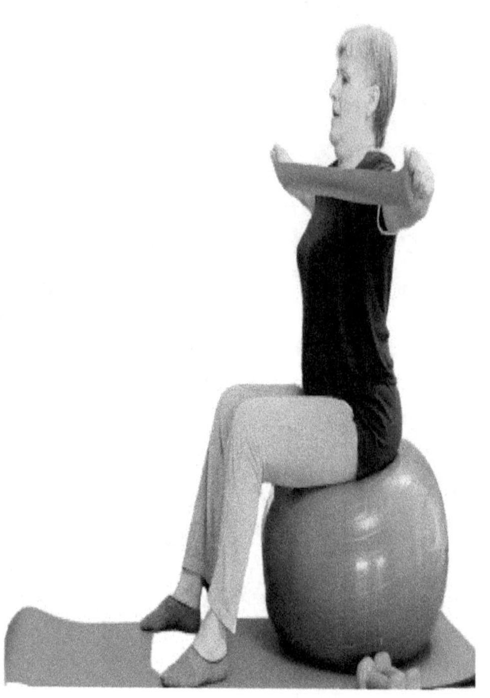